GUIDE TO NOOM DIET MEAL PLAN

LOSE WEIGHT AND GET FIT

Thomas M. Cook

Disclaimer

This publication is designed to provide competent and reliable information regarding the subject covered. However, the views expressed in this publication are those of the author alone, and should not be taken as expert instruction or professional advice. The reader is responsible for his or her actions. The author hereby disclaims any responsibility or liability whatsoever that is incurred from the use or application of the contents of this publication by the purchaser of the reader. The purchaser or reader is hereby responsible for his or her actions.

Table of Contents

INTRODUCTION

The Noom diet is a personalized weight loss plan that can be accessed through a phone app of the same name. According to the app's creators, it helps people reach their personal weight goals.

Customers of the Noom app can access a health consultant as well as a personalized nutrition plan.

People can also use the app to track their diet and exercise habits, as well as share their weight-loss success stories on Noom's social network.

Noom, a healthcare technology app, may be a good fit for you if you enjoy smartphone apps and virtual engagement. With Noom, it's not so much about what you eat as it is about why you eat. Noom encourages self-awareness, accountability, and the development of behaviors that can lead to weight loss and the maintenance of a healthy body weight.

On the Noom Healthy Weight app, you record every meal and snack, as well as your daily weight and exercise. Your one-on-one coach interacts with you and offers encouragement via the app's chat feature. You also communicate with your Noom group therapy coach and the other members of your chosen group.

DEFINITION OF NOOM

Noom is a diet and exercise program created by behavioral psychologists, dietitians, and personal trainers. It claims to be more interested in enacting concrete, long-term lifestyle changes than in encouraging more extreme eating habits (e.g., cutting out certain food groups or nutrients). The app, which Noom claims is the #1 scientifically proven sustainable weight-loss strategy, lets you do the following:

Create a personalized calorie breakdown using a series of lifestyle questions.

To keep track of what you eat, use a website or scan barcodes.

Keep track of your physical activity, weight, blood pressure, and blood glucose levels.

You can receive one-on-one health coaching in-app during business hours.

Keep yourself motivated by reading interesting articles and taking quizzes.

According to Noom, the coaching and material are designed to "help you obtain specialized information, tools, and abilities that can help you modify your habits, reduce weight, and make real progress well beyond scale." They also claim that people who use the Noom app and live a healthy lifestyle lose 15.5 pounds in 16 weeks on average.

IS NOOM EXPENSIVE?

A free trial may be provided depending on the time of year, but the Noom program generally starts at $60/month. Lower prices result from longer subscriptions. Noom's most affordable option is the yearly auto-recurring plan, which costs $199 (a little more than $16 per month). While users previously complained that it was difficult to cancel after a free trial, Noom appears to have simplified the process; you can cancel under the Settings section of the Manage Subscription tab. We were able to cancel our subscription through iTunes subscriptions on our smartphone because we purchased it through Apple.

ADVANTAGE OF NOON DIET

Our nutritionists appreciate that Noom concentrates on lifestyle modifications and the development of long-term healthy habits rather than advertising easy solutions with weight-loss smoothies and pills. You don't have to give up any meals, and Noom also promotes vital health and wellness principles like getting enough sleep and learning coping skills to deal with stress. One of the first mini classes you take asks you to step back and analyze potential

9

barriers to sticking to your goals, as well as to understand the factors that influence your eating choices in the present.

The app also encourages the consumption of real, whole foods and suggests eating more nutritious meals and snacks as frequently as possible. An algorithm calculates your individual energy needs and asks you to report what you eat, an evidence-based strategy that keeps you in touch with how much you eat and what types of foods you prefer. We were pleased to see that the food database included dishes from meal-delivery services such as Daily Harvest and Hello Fresh for easy tracking. You can also scan the barcode on packed items for real-time feedback while grocery shopping.

DISADVANTAGE OF NOOM DIET

Noom used to proclaim that it is not a diet, but lets be clear: Noom is a diet, plain and simple. Noom, or any other diet in general, is not recommended if you have a history of dieting. Noom appears to have improved since getting criticism, including now inquiring about any background of eating disorders and realigning the calorie levels to be less strict.

The program's color-coded meal system based on caloric density is our experts' favourite things gripe. This isn't a new concept and has been used in different diet plans in various ways in the past. Noom divides its groups as follows:

Green foods have the fewest calories and/or the greatest concentration of healthful nutrients. Several vegetables, fruits, egg whites, tofu, shrimp, nonfat milk and nonfat dairy products, and other foods are examples.

Yellow foods have more calories per serving and/or less healthful nutrients than green ones. Avocado, salmon, lean ground beef, black beans, olives, hummus, and other ingredients are among them.

Red foods are the most caloric intake and/or have the fewest healthful nutrients. Full-fat milk products, nut and seed butters, uncoated rice cakes, and other items are examples.

The colors, according to Noom, do not represent good or bad dishes, but rather serve as a portion recommendation. According to our experts, most people struggle to associate green meals with "healthy" foods and yellow and red meals with "poor" foods. Others may develop unhealthy food relationships and associations as a result of this, which is important to be aware of before beginning the program.

Furthermore, our certified dietitians were perplexed by a few of the food color classifications. Quinoa and eggs are considered yellow foods, whereas ultra-processed nonfat cheeses are considered green. Green foods may have fewer calories, but they may not be the healthiest, which is far more important than any number on the scale. In the opinion of our nutritionists, vilifying some of the world's best foods, such as avocados, chickpeas, almonds, and flax seeds (mentioned as red on Noom's system), isn't a long-term way to improve health. To Noom's credit, they provide a reasonable limit for each color-coded category and explicitly state that the majority of your diet will not consist of green items, which is fine.

The minimum monthly fee of $60 is quite high for a weight-loss app, and one of the most common online complaints is whether the app is "worth it." In comparison, WW (formerly Weight Watchers) offers a variety of areas of study, with their top-tier program providing personal coaching and virtual capabilities and costing roughly the same. Other health apps (such as MyFitnessPal) provide similar food tracking features for free to help people form healthier habits. Furthermore, recent Duke University research on free apps that allow people to track their progress discovered that whether you pay for a service or not may make no difference.

Noom might not be right for you if you need more structure, such as a well-planned meal plan. While Noom provides advice in the form of measurements and recipes, it does not provide a personalized food plan. Creating your own regular menu and planning meals for the week allows you more flexibility, but some people work much better with a much more regimented approach, so it all depends on your personal preferences. Of course, before beginning any new weight-loss or physiological program, consult with your doctor.

WILL NOOM ASSIST YOU IN LOSING WEIGHT?

To help you lose weight, most diets eliminate certain foods, such as carbs, calories, sugar, or fat. Noom is unique. It's a diet app that employs a psychological approach to changing your eating habits for the better. Noom's website claims that it uses technology to "help you change not just how you eat, but how you think."

Examining why you eat what you eat and making changes isn't a novel concept. However, the convenience of an app is crucial in this case. That strategy could explain why Noom has received over 50 million downloads since its debut in 2013.

Noom's Healthy Weight Program is a comprehensive wellness program that includes food, exercise, and mental health components. The goal is to alter your behavior so that you not only lose weight but also keep it off in the long run.

To begin, download the app and enter your height, weight, gender, age, general health information, goal weight, social circles, and other details about your life. Then, every day, you record your meals and snacks. The app provides feedback on your food choices to help you eat better and reach your weight-loss goals.

Noom's Healthy Weight Program is a comprehensive wellness program that includes food, exercise, and mental health components. The goal is to alter your behavior so that you not only lose weight but also keep it off in the long run.

To begin, download the app and enter your height, weight, gender, age, general health information, goal weight, social circles, and other details about your life. Then, every day, you record your meals and snacks. The app provides feedback on your food choices to help you eat better and reach your weight-loss goals.

In May 2018, a study published in the Journal of Nutrition compared weight loss with a low-calorie-dense diet to unrestrained eating in over 100 obese or overweight women in the United Kingdom. Those who followed low-calorie-dense diets lost more weight and reported fewer cravings over the course of the 12-week study.

A meta-analysis of 13 published studies in the April 2016 issue of Nutrients confirmed the link between low-density diets and weight loss.

A subsequent study, published in the European Journal of Nutrition in October 2016, examined the eating habits of more than 9,500 people. People who ate a higher proportion of low- and very-low-calorie-dense meals had lower body mass indexes (or BMI, which takes into account both weight and height) and smaller waist sizes. and are much less likely to be obese.

New research backs up some of the Noom components:

According to a recent Noom study, a food-categorization system, specifically Noom's color-coding, imparts health and nutrition knowledge that becomes unavoidable and allows people to maintain a healthier diet for up to 18 months. The findings were published in the journal Nutrients in May 2021.

According to a 2020 study, technology-based weight loss therapies are most effective when human comments and assistance are included.

According to the Noom website, those who complete the program lose 7.5

percent of their body weight on average, with 60 percent of users maintaining their weight loss one year later.

A number of studies are available on the Noom website to support the plan's weight-loss effectiveness. Many of those papers, however, have Noom team members among the writers.

Noom and independent studies both demonstrate the utility of smartphone apps in maintaining and promoting behavioural changes among motivated individuals.

HOW MUCH WORKOUT SHOULD YOU GET?

Exercise – and simply getting you to move more – is another everyday behavioral change that Noom encourages. Noom tracks your walking by counting your steps with your smartphone's built-in motion sensor. When you're ready, you can increase your step count. Running and other fitness activities may also be tracked by the software.

RISK ASSOCIATED TO NOOM DIET

The Noom app has a drawback in that users cannot collect data on components other than calories. A nutritious, well-balanced diet, on the other hand, should contain an adequate amount of nutrients such as vitamins and minerals.

As a result of this limitation, Noom app users will lack information about the nutritional composition and potential health benefits of their meal choices. It also suggests that doctors and nutritionists may be hesitant to recommend the app.

Furthermore, some Noom coaches are not National Board for Health and Wellness Coaching certified. This standard requires a coach to have the bare minimum of health and wellness coaching skills and knowledge.

Coaches who do not hold this certification may provide incorrect advice.

It is critical to emphasize that people with a complicated medical history should exercise extreme caution when using Noom or similar weight loss apps. Individuals in this category should seek additional weight loss advice from a doctor, dietician, or other healthcare professional.

CONCLUSION

Because Noom encourages habit development and the behavior-change-for-life tools used to assist guide you have some actual, considerable benefits, it may be good to start with the trial period.

However, your achievement on Noom will eventually be determined by how consistently you adhere to the program, use their coaches, and start engaging with their regular content. If the app's content or coaching programs make you feel ashamed or unworthy for any reason, it's time to unsubscribe. The same is true if you discover that the color-coded system promotes unhealthy food connections and anything other than limits and balanced eating. Using apps for monitoring may be beneficial for some people, but it does not guarantee that it will work for everyone, especially since improving your health and losing weight is highly dependent on your individual preferences and goals. On a paid platform, it may be difficult to distinguish what works for you from what appears to work for everyone else. Improved health and weight loss require you to take control of the changes you make – within the boundaries of your own unique emotional, physical, and psychological boundaries. Remember that, and you'll be well on your way to long-term success.

Printed in Great Britain
by Amazon

43970665R00020